Planner

....

MONTH -
To Do List -
- [ ]
- [ ]
- [ ]
- [ ]
- [ ]
- [ ]
- [ ]

Monday -

Tuesday -

Wednesday -

Thursday -

Friday -

Saturday -

Sunday -

Notes -

MONTH -
To Do List -
- [ ]
- [ ]
- [ ]
- [ ]
- [ ]
- [ ]
- [ ]

Monday -

Tuesday -

Wednesday -

Thursday -

Friday -

Saturday -

Sunday -

Notes -

MONTH -
To Do List -

Monday -

Tuesday -

Wednesday -

Thursday -

Friday -

Saturday -

Sunday -

Notes -

MONTH -
To Do List -

- [ ]
- [ ]
- [ ]
- [ ]
- [ ]
- [ ]
- [ ]

Monday -

Tuesday -

Wednesday -

Thursday -

Friday -

Saturday -

Sunday -

Notes -

MONTH -
To Do List -

- [ ]
- [ ]
- [ ]
- [ ]
- [ ]
- [ ]
- [ ]

Monday -

Tuesday -

Wednesday -

Thursday -

Friday -

Saturday -

Sunday -

Notes -

MONTH -
To Do List -
- [ ]
- [ ]
- [ ]
- [ ]
- [ ]
- [ ]
- [ ]

Monday -

Tuesday -

Wednesday -

Thursday -

Friday -

Saturday -

Sunday -

Notes -

MONTH -
To Do List -
- [ ]
- [ ]
- [ ]
- [ ]
- [ ]
- [ ]
- [ ]

Monday -

Tuesday -

Wednesday -

Thursday -

Friday -

Saturday -

Sunday -

Notes -

MONTH -
To Do List -

- ☐
- ☐
- ☐
- ☐
- ☐
- ☐
- ☐

Monday -

Tuesday -

Wednesday -

Thursday -

Friday -

Saturday -

Sunday -

Notes -

MONTH -

To Do List -

- [ ]
- [ ]
- [ ]
- [ ]
- [ ]
- [ ]
- [ ]

Monday -

Tuesday -

Wednesday -

Thursday -

Friday -

Saturday -

Sunday -

Notes -

MONTH -
To Do List -

- [ ]
- [ ]
- [ ]
- [ ]
- [ ]
- [ ]
- [ ]

Monday -

Tuesday -

Wednesday -

Thursday -

Friday -

Saturday -

Sunday -

Notes -

MONTH -
To Do List -
- [ ]
- [ ]
- [ ]
- [ ]
- [ ]
- [ ]
- [ ]

Monday -

Tuesday -

Wednesday -

Thursday -

Friday -

Saturday -

Sunday -

Notes -

MONTH -
To Do List -
- [ ]
- [ ]
- [ ]
- [ ]
- [ ]
- [ ]
- [ ]

Monday -

Tuesday -

Wednesday -

Thursday -

Friday -

Saturday -

Sunday -

Notes -

MONTH -
To Do List -

- [ ]
- [ ]
- [ ]
- [ ]
- [ ]
- [ ]
- [ ]

Monday -

Tuesday -

Wednesday -

Thursday -

Friday -

Saturday -

Sunday -

Notes -

MONTH -

To Do List -

- [ ]
- [ ]
- [ ]
- [ ]
- [ ]
- [ ]
- [ ]

Monday -

Tuesday -

Wednesday -

Thursday -

Friday -

Saturday -

Sunday -

Notes -

MONTH -
To Do List -

- [ ]
- [ ]
- [ ]
- [ ]
- [ ]
- [ ]
- [ ]

Monday -

Tuesday -

Wednesday -

Thursday -

Friday -

Saturday -

Sunday -

Notes -

MONTH -
To Do List -

- [ ]
- [ ]
- [ ]
- [ ]
- [ ]
- [ ]
- [ ]

Monday -

Tuesday -

Wednesday -

Thursday -

Friday -

Saturday -

Sunday -

Notes -

MONTH -
To Do List -
- [ ]
- [ ]
- [ ]
- [ ]
- [ ]
- [ ]
- [ ]

Monday -

Tuesday -

Wednesday -

Thursday -

Friday -

Saturday -

Sunday -

Notes -

MONTH -

To Do List -

- [ ]
- [ ]
- [ ]
- [ ]
- [ ]
- [ ]
- [ ]

Monday -

Tuesday -

Wednesday -

Thursday -

Friday -

Saturday -

Sunday -

Notes -

MONTH -

To Do List -

- [ ]
- [ ]
- [ ]
- [ ]
- [ ]
- [ ]
- [ ]

Monday -

Tuesday -

Wednesday -

Thursday -

Friday -

Saturday -

Sunday -

Notes -

MONTH -
To Do List -
- [ ]
- [ ]
- [ ]
- [ ]
- [ ]
- [ ]
- [ ]

Monday -

Tuesday -

Wednesday -

Thursday -

Friday -

Saturday -

Sunday -

Notes -

MONTH -
To Do List -

- [ ]
- [ ]
- [ ]
- [ ]
- [ ]
- [ ]
- [ ]

Monday -

Tuesday -

Wednesday -

Thursday -

Friday -

Saturday -

Sunday -

Notes -

MONTH -

To Do List -

- [ ]
- [ ]
- [ ]
- [ ]
- [ ]
- [ ]
- [ ]

Monday -

Tuesday -

Wednesday -

Thursday -

Friday -

Saturday -

Sunday -

Notes -

MONTH -
To Do List -

- [ ]
- [ ]
- [ ]
- [ ]
- [ ]
- [ ]
- [ ]

Monday -

Tuesday -

Wednesday -

Thursday -

Friday -

Saturday -

Sunday -

Notes -

MONTH -
To Do List -

- [ ]
- [ ]
- [ ]
- [ ]
- [ ]
- [ ]
- [ ]

Monday -

Tuesday -

Wednesday -

Thursday -

Friday -

Saturday -

Sunday -

Notes -

MONTH -
To Do List -
- [ ]
- [ ]
- [ ]
- [ ]
- [ ]
- [ ]
- [ ]

Monday -

Tuesday -

Wednesday -

Thursday -

Friday -

Saturday -

Sunday -

Notes -

MONTH -
To Do List -

- [ ]
- [ ]
- [ ]
- [ ]
- [ ]
- [ ]
- [ ]

Monday -

Tuesday -

Wednesday -

Thursday -

Friday -

Saturday -

Sunday -

Notes -

MONTH -
To Do List -

- [ ]
- [ ]
- [ ]
- [ ]
- [ ]
- [ ]
- [ ]

Monday -

Tuesday -

Wednesday -

Thursday -

Friday -

Saturday -

Sunday -

Notes -

MONTH -
To Do List -
- [ ]
- [ ]
- [ ]
- [ ]
- [ ]
- [ ]
- [ ]

Monday -

Tuesday -

Wednesday -

Thursday -

Friday -

Saturday -

Sunday -

Notes -

MONTH -
To Do List -

- [ ]
- [ ]
- [ ]
- [ ]
- [ ]
- [ ]
- [ ]

Monday -

Tuesday -

Wednesday -

Thursday -

Friday -

Saturday -

Sunday -

Notes -

MONTH -
To Do List -

- [ ]
- [ ]
- [ ]
- [ ]
- [ ]
- [ ]
- [ ]

Monday -

Tuesday -

Wednesday -

Thursday -

Friday -

Saturday -

Sunday -

Notes -

MONTH -
To Do List -
- [ ]
- [ ]
- [ ]
- [ ]
- [ ]
- [ ]
- [ ]

Monday -

Tuesday -

Wednesday -

Thursday -

Friday -

Saturday -

Sunday -

Notes -

MONTH -
To Do List -

- [ ]
- [ ]
- [ ]
- [ ]
- [ ]
- [ ]
- [ ]

Monday -

Tuesday -

Wednesday -

Thursday -

Friday -

Saturday -

Sunday -

Notes -

MONTH -

To Do List -

- [ ]
- [ ]
- [ ]
- [ ]
- [ ]
- [ ]
- [ ]

Monday -

Tuesday -

Wednesday -

Thursday -

Friday -

Saturday -

Sunday -

Notes -

MONTH -
To Do List -

- [ ]
- [ ]
- [ ]
- [ ]
- [ ]
- [ ]
- [ ]

Monday -

Tuesday -

Wednesday -

Thursday -

Friday -

Saturday -

Sunday -

Notes -

MONTH -
To Do List -
- [ ]
- [ ]
- [ ]
- [ ]
- [ ]
- [ ]
- [ ]

Monday -

Tuesday -

Wednesday -

Thursday -

Friday -

Saturday -

Sunday -

Notes -

MONTH -
To Do List -

- [ ]
- [ ]
- [ ]
- [ ]
- [ ]
- [ ]
- [ ]

Monday -

Tuesday -

Wednesday -

Thursday -

Friday -

Saturday -

Sunday -

Notes -

MONTH -

To Do List -

- [ ]
- [ ]
- [ ]
- [ ]
- [ ]
- [ ]
- [ ]

Monday -

Tuesday -

Wednesday -

Thursday -

Friday -

Saturday -

Sunday -

Notes -

MONTH -
To Do List -
- [ ]
- [ ]
- [ ]
- [ ]
- [ ]
- [ ]
- [ ]

Monday -

Tuesday -

Wednesday -

Thursday -

Friday -

Saturday -

Sunday -

Notes -

MONTH -

To Do List -
- [ ]
- [ ]
- [ ]
- [ ]
- [ ]
- [ ]
- [ ]

Monday -

Tuesday -

Wednesday -

Thursday -

Friday -

Saturday -

Sunday -

Notes -

MONTH -
To Do List -

- [ ]
- [ ]
- [ ]
- [ ]
- [ ]
- [ ]
- [ ]

Monday -

Tuesday -

Wednesday -

Thursday -

Friday -

Saturday -

Sunday -

Notes -

MONTH -
To Do List -

- [ ]
- [ ]
- [ ]
- [ ]
- [ ]
- [ ]
- [ ]

Monday -

Tuesday -

Wednesday -

Thursday -

Friday -

Saturday -

Sunday -

Notes -

MONTH -
To Do List -
- [ ]
- [ ]
- [ ]
- [ ]
- [ ]
- [ ]
- [ ]

Monday -

Tuesday -

Wednesday -

Thursday -

Friday -

Saturday -

Sunday -

Notes -

MONTH -
To Do List -

- [ ]
- [ ]
- [ ]
- [ ]
- [ ]
- [ ]
- [ ]

Monday -

Tuesday -

Wednesday -

Thursday -

Friday -

Saturday -

Sunday -

Notes -

MONTH -

To Do List -

- [ ]
- [ ]
- [ ]
- [ ]
- [ ]
- [ ]
- [ ]

Monday -

Tuesday -

Wednesday -

Thursday -

Friday -

Saturday -

Sunday -

Notes -

MONTH -

To Do List -

- [ ]
- [ ]
- [ ]
- [ ]
- [ ]
- [ ]
- [ ]

Monday -

Tuesday -

Wednesday -

Thursday -

Friday -

Saturday -

Sunday -

Notes -

MONTH -
To Do List -

- [ ]
- [ ]
- [ ]
- [ ]
- [ ]
- [ ]
- [ ]

Monday -

Tuesday -

Wednesday -

Thursday -

Friday -

Saturday -

Sunday -

Notes -

MONTH -
To Do List -
- [ ]
- [ ]
- [ ]
- [ ]
- [ ]
- [ ]
- [ ]

Monday -

Tuesday -

Wednesday -

Thursday -

Friday -

Saturday -

Sunday -

Notes -

MONTH -
To Do List -
- [ ]
- [ ]
- [ ]
- [ ]
- [ ]
- [ ]
- [ ]

Monday -

Tuesday -

Wednesday -

Thursday -

Friday -

Saturday -

Sunday -

Notes -

MONTH -

To Do List -

- [ ]
- [ ]
- [ ]
- [ ]
- [ ]
- [ ]
- [ ]

Monday -

Tuesday -

Wednesday -

Thursday -

Friday -

Saturday -

Sunday -

Notes -

MONTH -
To Do List -

- [ ]
- [ ]
- [ ]
- [ ]
- [ ]
- [ ]
- [ ]

Monday -

Tuesday -

Wednesday -

Thursday -

Friday -

Saturday -

Sunday -

Notes -

MONTH -
To Do List -
- [ ]
- [ ]
- [ ]
- [ ]
- [ ]
- [ ]
- [ ]

Monday -

Tuesday -

Wednesday -

Thursday -

Friday -

Saturday -

Sunday -

Notes -

MONTH -

To Do List -
- [ ]
- [ ]
- [ ]
- [ ]
- [ ]
- [ ]
- [ ]

Monday -

Tuesday -

Wednesday -

Thursday -

Friday -

Saturday -

Sunday -

Notes -

MONTH -
To Do List -

- ☐
- ☐
- ☐
- ☐
- ☐
- ☐
- ☐

Monday -

Tuesday -

Wednesday -

Thursday -

Friday -

Saturday -

Sunday -

Notes -

MONTH -

To Do List -

- [ ]
- [ ]
- [ ]
- [ ]
- [ ]
- [ ]
- [ ]

Monday -

Tuesday -

Wednesday -

Thursday -

Friday -

Saturday -

Sunday -

Notes -

MONTH -
To Do List -

- [ ]
- [ ]
- [ ]
- [ ]
- [ ]
- [ ]
- [ ]

Monday -

Tuesday -

Wednesday -

Thursday -

Friday -

Saturday -

Sunday -

Notes -

MONTH -
To Do List -

- [ ]
- [ ]
- [ ]
- [ ]
- [ ]
- [ ]
- [ ]

Monday -

Tuesday -

Wednesday -

Thursday -

Friday -

Saturday -

Sunday -

Notes -

MONTH -
To Do List -

- [ ]
- [ ]
- [ ]
- [ ]
- [ ]
- [ ]
- [ ]

Monday -

Tuesday -

Wednesday -

Thursday -

Friday -

Saturday -

Sunday -

Notes -

MONTH -
To Do List -

- [ ]
- [ ]
- [ ]
- [ ]
- [ ]
- [ ]
- [ ]

Monday -

Tuesday -

Wednesday -

Thursday -

Friday -

Saturday -

Sunday -

Notes -

MONTH -

To Do List -

- [ ]
- [ ]
- [ ]
- [ ]
- [ ]
- [ ]
- [ ]

Monday -

Tuesday -

Wednesday -

Thursday -

Friday -

Saturday -

Sunday -

Notes -

MONTH -
To Do List -

- [ ]
- [ ]
- [ ]
- [ ]
- [ ]
- [ ]
- [ ]

Monday -

Tuesday -

Wednesday -

Thursday -

Friday -

Saturday -

Sunday -

Notes -

NAME	CONTACT DETAILS

NAME	CONTACT DETAILS

NAME	CONTACT DETAILS

NAME	CONTACT DETAILS

Company - Website	Passwords

Company - Website	Passwords

www.ingramcontent.com/pod-product-compliance
Lightning Source LLC
Chambersburg PA
CBHW062332220526
45469CB00008B/2687